THE AMANPURI DIET

The Best Strategy for Losing Weight and Managing Your Hormones

By

Donald V. Schaper

DISCLAIMER

TABLE OF CONTENT

CHAPTER ONE

INTRODUCTION

Losing weight can be a challenging task for many people, especially when it comes to keeping the weight off in the long run. However, what most people don't realize is that weight management is not just about eating less and exercising more. It is also about understanding the role of hormones in weight loss and adopting a lifestyle that supports hormonal balance. Hormonal imbalances can make it difficult to lose weight and maintain a healthy weight. Thus, managing hormones is crucial to achieving and maintaining a healthy weight. In this regard, the Amanpuri Diet has emerged as one of the best strategies for losing weight and managing hormones. This diet is based on the principles of whole foods, low-glycemic index foods, healthy fats, and adequate protein, which help balance hormones and promote weight loss.

Losing weight is a goal that many people strive to achieve. However, it is not always easy to lose weight and keep it off in the long run. One of the reasons why weight loss can be challenging is the role of hormones in weight management. Hormones play a crucial role in regulating various bodily functions, including metabolism and appetite. Therefore, any hormonal imbalances can significantly affect weight loss efforts. Hormonal imbalances can lead to issues such as insulin resistance, leptin resistance, and thyroid dysfunction, which can make it difficult to lose weight.

The Amanpuri Diet has gained popularity as one of the best strategies for losing weight and managing hormones. This diet is based on the principles of whole foods, low-glycemic index foods, healthy fats, and adequate protein, which help balance hormones and promote weight loss. The Amanpuri Diet encourages the consumption of whole, unprocessed foods such as fruits, vegetables, whole grains, and lean proteins. It emphasizes the importance of consuming low-glycemic index foods, which can help regulate blood sugar levels and prevent insulin spikes. The diet also emphasizes healthy fats such as those found in nuts, seeds, and avocados, which can help regulate hormones.

Moreover, the Amanpuri Diet is designed to help individuals manage their hormones through dietary and lifestyle changes. It focuses on eliminating processed foods, added sugars, and refined carbohydrates, which can lead to hormonal imbalances. The diet also emphasizes the importance of exercise, stress management, and getting adequate sleep, all of which can support hormonal balance.

The Amanpuri Diet offers a holistic approach to weight management by addressing the role of hormones in weight loss. By adopting the principles of the Amanpuri Diet, individuals can not only lose weight but also manage their hormones, leading to long-term success in maintaining a healthy weight.

CHAPTER TWO

Understanding Hormones and Weight Loss

Hormones play a significant role in regulating various bodily functions, including metabolism and appetite. Therefore, any hormonal imbalances can significantly affect weight loss efforts. Understanding the role of hormones in weight management is crucial to achieving and maintaining a healthy weight.

One of the key hormones involved in weight management is insulin. Insulin is a hormone produced by the pancreas that regulates blood sugar levels by promoting the uptake of glucose by cells. Insulin resistance, a condition in which the body becomes less responsive to insulin, can lead to elevated blood sugar levels, which can increase the risk of developing type 2 diabetes and obesity.

Another important hormone in weight management is leptin. Leptin is a hormone produced by fat cells that helps regulate energy balance by signaling the brain to reduce appetite and increase energy expenditure. Leptin resistance, a condition in which the body becomes less responsive to leptin, can lead to increased appetite and reduced energy expenditure, which can contribute to obesity.

Thyroid hormones also play a crucial role in weight management. Thyroid hormones regulate metabolism, which is the rate at which the body burns calories. Low levels of thyroid hormones can lead to a slower metabolism, making it more difficult to lose weight.

Cortisol, a hormone produced by the adrenal glands, also plays a role in weight management. Cortisol is often referred to as the "stress hormone" as it is released in response to stress. High levels of cortisol can lead to increased appetite, particularly for high-fat, high-sugar foods, which can contribute to weight gain.

Moreover, sex hormones such as estrogen and testosterone also play a role in weight management. In women, low levels of estrogen can lead to weight gain, particularly around the abdomen. In men, low levels of testosterone can lead to decreased muscle mass and increased body fat, which can contribute to weight gain.

The Amanpuri Diet is designed to help individuals manage their hormones through dietary and lifestyle changes. By adopting the principles of the Amanpuri Diet, individuals can regulate blood sugar levels, improve insulin sensitivity, and reduce the risk of insulin resistance. The diet also promotes the consumption of foods that are rich in nutrients that support hormonal balance, such as healthy fats and protein.

Understanding the role of hormones in weight management is crucial to achieving and maintaining a healthy weight. By adopting a diet and lifestyle that supports hormonal balance, individuals can achieve long-term success in managing their weight.

In addition to diet and lifestyle changes, other strategies can be used to support hormonal balance and weight management. For example, exercise has been shown to improve insulin sensitivity and reduce cortisol levels, both of which can help with weight loss. Resistance training, in particular, is effective in increasing muscle mass and improving insulin sensitivity, which can lead to long-term weight loss success.

Stress management techniques such as mindfulness meditation, yoga, and deep breathing can also be effective in reducing cortisol levels and improving overall hormonal balance. Getting adequate sleep is also essential as sleep deprivation can lead to hormonal imbalances that can contribute to weight gain.

Moreover, several supplements can be used to support hormonal balance and weight management. For example, omega-3 fatty acids, found in fish oil supplements, have been shown to reduce inflammation and improve insulin sensitivity, which can help with weight loss. Probiotic supplements can also be effective in improving gut health, which can support hormonal balance and weight loss.

Achieving and maintaining a healthy weight is not just about calorie counting and exercise. Understanding the role of hormones in weight management and adopting a holistic approach to weight loss that includes dietary and lifestyle changes, exercise, stress management, and adequate sleep can lead to long-term success in managing weight. Moreover, using supplements that support hormonal balance can also be effective in achieving weight loss goals.

Role of Hormones in Weight Management

Hormones play a crucial role in regulating various physiological processes, including metabolism, appetite, and energy balance. Therefore, any hormonal imbalances can significantly affect weight management efforts. Understanding the role of hormones in weight management is essential to achieving and maintaining a healthy weight.

Insulin is one of the key hormones involved in weight management. Insulin is a hormone produced by the pancreas that regulates blood sugar levels by promoting the uptake of glucose by cells. Insulin resistance, a condition in which the body becomes less responsive to insulin, can lead to elevated blood sugar levels, which can increase the risk of developing type 2 diabetes and obesity.

Leptin is another important hormone involved in weight management. Leptin is a hormone produced by fat cells that helps regulate energy balance by signaling the brain to reduce appetite and increase energy expenditure. Leptin resistance, a condition in which the body becomes less responsive to leptin, can lead to increased appetite and reduced energy expenditure, which can contribute to obesity.

Thyroid hormones also play a crucial role in weight management. Thyroid hormones regulate metabolism, which is the rate at which the body burns calories. Low levels of thyroid hormones can lead to a slower metabolism, making it more difficult to lose weight.

Cortisol, a hormone produced by the adrenal glands, also plays a role in weight management. Cortisol is often referred to as the "stress hormone" as it is released in response to stress. High levels of cortisol can lead to increased appetite, particularly for high-fat, high-sugar foods, which can contribute to weight gain.

Moreover, sex hormones such as estrogen and testosterone also play a role in weight management. In women, low levels of estrogen can lead to weight gain, particularly around the abdomen. In men, low levels of testosterone can lead to decreased muscle mass and increased body fat, which can contribute to weight gain.

To manage weight effectively, it is important to understand how these hormones work and how they can be influenced by diet and lifestyle choices. For example, adopting a diet that is rich in fiber, protein, and healthy fats can help regulate blood sugar levels, improve insulin sensitivity, and reduce the risk of insulin resistance.

Similarly, incorporating regular exercise into a daily routine can help regulate hormones such as cortisol and improve insulin sensitivity.

Additionally, stress management techniques such as meditation, yoga, and deep breathing can help reduce cortisol levels and improve overall hormonal balance. Getting adequate sleep is also essential as sleep deprivation can lead to hormonal imbalances that can contribute to weight gain.

Hormones play a significant role in weight management, and any imbalances can significantly affect weight loss efforts. Understanding the role of hormones in weight management and adopting a holistic approach that includes dietary and lifestyle changes, exercise, stress management, and adequate sleep can lead to long-term success in managing weight. Moreover, using supplements that support hormonal balance can also be effective in achieving weight loss goals.

In addition to the strategies mentioned above, there are other ways to support hormonal balance and weight management. For example, intermittent fasting has been shown to improve insulin sensitivity and reduce insulin resistance, which can lead to weight loss. Intermittent fasting involves restricting calorie intake to certain periods of the day, such as eating within an 8-hour window and fasting for the remaining 16 hours.

Moreover, dietary supplements can also be effective in supporting hormonal balance and weight management. For example, chromium picolinate is a supplement that has been shown to improve insulin sensitivity and reduce insulin resistance, which can lead to weight loss. Similarly, green tea extract contains compounds called catechins, which have been shown to increase metabolism and fat burning.

It is also important to note that hormonal imbalances can be caused by underlying health conditions, such as polycystic ovary syndrome (PCOS) and hypothyroidism. Therefore, it is important to consult a healthcare professional if hormonal imbalances are suspected, particularly if weight management efforts are not successful.

Furthermore, hormonal changes can also occur naturally during different stages of life, such as menopause. During menopause, estrogen levels decrease, which can lead to weight gain, particularly around the abdomen. Therefore, adopting a healthy lifestyle that includes regular exercise, a balanced diet, stress management, and adequate sleep can help manage weight during menopause.

Hormonal imbalances can significantly affect weight management efforts. Understanding the role of hormones in weight management and adopting a holistic approach that includes dietary and lifestyle changes, exercise, stress management, and adequate sleep can lead to long-term success in managing weight. Moreover, using supplements that support hormonal balance and consulting a healthcare professional if underlying health conditions are suspected can also be effective in achieving weight loss goals.

Common Hormonal Imbalances That Affect Weight

Several common hormonal imbalances can affect weight management efforts. These hormonal imbalances can be caused by various factors such as genetics, lifestyle, diet, and underlying health conditions. Understanding these imbalances is essential for effective weight management.

For example, lifestyle factors such as diet, exercise, stress, and sleep can play a significant role in hormonal balance and weight management. A diet high in processed and sugary foods can contribute to insulin resistance and leptin resistance. Regular exercise can help improve insulin sensitivity and reduce cortisol levels, while adequate sleep can help regulate hormone levels and support weight management efforts.

Additionally, underlying health conditions such as PCOS and hypothyroidism can also contribute to hormonal imbalances and weight gain. These conditions require medical management, and it is essential to consult a healthcare professional for proper diagnosis and treatment.

It is also important to note that hormonal imbalances can affect individuals differently. For example, some people may experience significant weight gain with PCOS, while others may not. Similarly, the same hormonal imbalance may affect different individuals in different ways, depending on their genetics, lifestyle, and overall health.

Insulin Resistance

Insulin resistance is a common hormonal imbalance that can affect weight management. It is a condition in which the body becomes less responsive to insulin, a hormone that regulates blood sugar levels. Insulin resistance can lead to elevated blood sugar levels, which can increase the risk of developing type 2 diabetes and obesity. High levels of insulin also lead to the body storing more fat, particularly around the abdomen.

Leptin Resistance

Leptin is a hormone produced by fat cells that helps regulate energy balance by signaling the brain to reduce appetite and increase energy expenditure. Leptin resistance is a condition in which the body becomes less responsive to leptin. It can lead to increased appetite and reduced energy expenditure, which can contribute to obesity.

Thyroid Hormone Imbalance

The thyroid gland produces hormones that regulate metabolism, the rate at which the body burns calories. An underactive thyroid gland (hypothyroidism) can lead to a slower metabolism, making it more difficult to lose weight. Conversely, an overactive thyroid gland (hyperthyroidism) can lead to a faster metabolism, making it difficult to gain weight.

Cortisol Imbalance

Cortisol is a hormone produced by the adrenal glands that is often referred to as the "stress hormone." It is released in response to stress and can lead to increased appetite, particularly for high-fat, high-sugar foods, which can contribute to weight gain.

Sex Hormone Imbalances

Sex hormones such as estrogen and testosterone play a role in weight management. In women, low levels of estrogen can lead to weight gain, particularly around the abdomen. In men, low levels of testosterone can lead to decreased muscle mass and increased body fat, which can contribute to weight gain.

Growth Hormone Imbalance

Growth hormone is a hormone produced by the pituitary gland that helps regulate metabolism and muscle growth. A deficiency in growth hormone can lead to decreased muscle mass and increased body fat, which can contribute to weight gain.

Polycystic Ovary Syndrome (PCOS)

PCOS is a common hormonal disorder that affects women of reproductive age. It is characterized by high levels of androgens (male hormones) and insulin resistance. These hormonal imbalances can lead to weight gain, particularly around the abdomen, and difficulty losing weight.

Menopause

During menopause, estrogen levels decrease, which can lead to weight gain, particularly around the abdomen. This hormonal change can make it more difficult to lose weight.

Hormonal imbalances can significantly affect weight management efforts. Understanding the common hormonal imbalances that can affect weight and their underlying causes can help individuals take steps to manage their weight effectively. Consulting a healthcare professional and adopting a healthy lifestyle that includes regular exercise, a balanced diet, stress management, and adequate sleep can help manage hormonal imbalances and support long-term weight management goals.

Therefore, the best approach to managing hormonal imbalances and weight is a personalized one. Individuals should consult with their healthcare professionals to determine the underlying causes of their hormonal imbalances and develop a personalized plan to manage their weight and support hormonal balance. This plan may include dietary changes, exercise, stress management, supplements, and medication, depending on the individual's unique needs.

Understanding the common hormonal imbalances that affect weight management, their underlying causes, and controllable factors such as lifestyle and diet, is essential for effective weight management. Consulting a healthcare professional and developing a personalized plan to manage hormonal imbalances can lead to long-term success in weight management and overall health.

How Diet Helps Balance Hormones

Hormones are the body's chemical messengers that regulate various functions in the body, including metabolism, growth and development, mood, and reproduction. Hormones work in harmony with each other, but any disruption in this balance can lead to health problems such as weight gain, mood swings, and infertility. Diet plays a crucial role in maintaining hormonal balance, and making the right dietary choices can help improve hormonal imbalances.

Here are some ways that diet helps balance hormones:

1. Control Insulin Levels: Insulin is a hormone that regulates blood sugar levels in the body. High insulin levels can lead to insulin resistance, which is a risk factor for type 2 diabetes, PCOS, and other hormonal imbalances. A diet that is high in refined carbohydrates and sugar can lead to insulin resistance, so it's essential to eat a balanced diet that includes complex carbohydrates, healthy fats, and protein. Eating fiber-rich foods such as vegetables, fruits, whole grains, and legumes can help regulate insulin levels.

2. Increase Fiber Intake: Fiber is an essential nutrient that helps regulate digestion and bowel movements. It also plays a crucial role in balancing hormones by binding to excess estrogen and helping to eliminate it from the body. Eating a diet rich in fiber can help prevent estrogen dominance and reduce the risk of breast cancer and other hormonal imbalances.

3. Choose Healthy Fats: Healthy fats such as omega-3 fatty acids and monounsaturated fats can help balance hormones. Omega-3 fatty acids are found in fatty fish, walnuts, chia seeds, and flaxseeds. These healthy fats can help reduce inflammation, improve insulin sensitivity, and balance hormones. Monounsaturated fats are found in foods such as avocado, olive oil, and nuts, and can help regulate hormones such as estrogen.

4. Avoid Processed Foods: Processed foods are often high in sugar, refined carbohydrates, and unhealthy fats.

These foods can disrupt hormonal balance and lead to insulin resistance, inflammation, and weight gain. Avoiding processed foods and eating whole, nutrient-dense foods can help balance hormones and improve overall health.

5. Increase Protein Intake: Protein is essential for building and repairing tissues in the body. It also plays a crucial role in balancing hormones, as some hormones such as insulin and growth hormone are made from protein. Eating a diet rich in protein can help regulate blood sugar levels, increase satiety, and improve insulin sensitivity. Good sources of protein include lean meats, fish, eggs, and plant-based options such as beans, lentils, and tofu.

6. **Include Phytoestrogens:** Phytoestrogens are plant-based compounds that mimic the effects of estrogen in the body. These compounds can help balance hormones by binding to estrogen receptors and regulating estrogen levels. Good sources of phytoestrogens include soy products such as tofu, tempeh, and edamame, as well as flaxseeds, sesame seeds, and legumes.

7. **Stay Hydrated:** Staying hydrated is essential for overall health and hormonal balance. Dehydration can lead to hormonal imbalances, as the body needs water to produce hormones. Drinking enough water can also help regulate digestion, metabolism, and blood sugar levels, which are all important factors in hormonal balance.

Diet plays a crucial role in balancing hormones, and making the right dietary choices can help improve hormonal imbalances. Eating a diet rich in fiber, healthy fats, protein, and phytoestrogens, while avoiding processed foods, can help regulate blood sugar levels, reduce inflammation, and balance hormones. Staying hydrated is also essential for hormonal balance, so it's important to drink enough water throughout the day.

CHAPTER THREE

Key Principles of the Amanpuri Diet

The Amanpuri Diet is a healthy eating plan that was created by the Amanpuri wellness resort in Phuket, Thailand. This diet emphasizes eating whole, nutrient-dense foods and avoiding processed and refined foods. The Amanpuri Diet is based on the principles of a balanced and sustainable lifestyle that promotes overall health and well-being. Here are the key principles of the Amanpuri Diet:

Eat Whole, Nutrient-Dense Foods: The Amanpuri Diet emphasizes eating whole foods that are nutrient-dense and minimally processed. This includes fresh fruits and vegetables, whole grains, lean proteins, and healthy fats such as nuts, seeds, and avocado. These foods are rich in vitamins, minerals, fiber, and antioxidants, which are essential for maintaining good health.

Avoid Processed and Refined Foods: The Amanpuri Diet discourages the consumption of processed and refined foods, such as white bread, pasta, and sugar. These foods are often stripped of their nutrients and can contribute to weight gain, inflammation, and other health problems. Instead, the diet encourages the consumption of whole grains and natural sweeteners, such as honey and maple syrup.

- **Balance Macronutrients:** The Amanpuri Diet focuses on balancing macronutrients, which are carbohydrates, proteins, and fats. The diet recommends consuming a balance of all three macronutrients at each meal to promote satiety, stabilize blood sugar levels, and maintain energy throughout the day. The recommended balance is 40% carbohydrates, 30% protein, and 30% healthy fats.

⊠ **Eat Mindfully:** The Amanpuri Diet emphasizes the importance of mindful eating, which involves paying attention to your body's hunger and fullness cues and eating slowly and consciously. This helps prevent overeating, promotes digestion, and allows for a greater appreciation of the food being consumed.

* **Emphasize Local and Seasonal Foods:** The Amanpuri Diet promotes the consumption of local and seasonal foods, which are fresher, more nutritious, and better for the environment. Eating locally and seasonally also supports local farmers and helps reduce the carbon footprint associated with transporting food over long distances.

- ⊠ **Hydrate Well:** The Amanpuri Diet stresses the importance of staying hydrated by drinking plenty of water throughout the day. Drinking enough water can help regulate digestion, metabolism, and blood sugar levels, and prevent dehydration, which can lead to hormonal imbalances.

- ⊠ **Listen to Your Body:** The Amanpuri Diet encourages individuals to listen to their bodies and make adjustments to their eating habits accordingly. This means paying attention to how different foods make you feel and making choices that support your overall health and well-being.

☒ **Incorporate Fermented Foods:** The Amanpuri Diet encourages the consumption of fermented foods, such as kefir, yogurt, kimchi, and sauerkraut. These foods are rich in probiotics, which promote gut health and aid in digestion. Incorporating fermented foods into your diet can help balance the microbiome in your gut, which can improve your overall health.

- ⊠ **Limit Alcohol Consumption:** The Amanpuri Diet recommends limiting alcohol consumption, as excessive drinking can lead to inflammation, liver damage, and hormonal imbalances. The diet suggests consuming alcohol in moderation and choosing lower calorie, lower sugar options such as wine or spirits mixed with soda water and fresh lime.

☒ **Practice Intermittent Fasting:** The Amanpuri Diet recommends practicing intermittent fasting, which involves alternating periods of eating and fasting. This can help improve insulin sensitivity, promote weight loss, and reduce inflammation in the body. The diet suggests starting with a 12-hour fast and gradually increasing the fasting window to up to 16 hours per day.

☒ **Support Sustainable Practices:** The Amanpuri Diet promotes sustainability by encouraging individuals to choose foods that are grown and harvested in an environmentally friendly way. This means choosing organic and sustainably farmed produce and meat and minimizing food waste by using leftovers and composting.

⊠ **Incorporate Movement and Mindfulness: The Amanpuri Diet recognizes** the importance of movement and mindfulness in promoting overall health and well-being. The diet encourages individuals to incorporate daily movement and exercise, such as yoga, walking, or swimming, and to practice mindfulness techniques such as meditation and deep breathing to reduce stress and improve mental health.

Overall, the Amanpuri Diet is a comprehensive approach to healthy eating that emphasizes the consumption of whole, nutrient-dense foods and the avoidance of processed and refined foods. The diet promotes balance, sustainability, and mindfulness in all aspects of eating and lifestyle habits, which can lead to improved overall health and well-being. By following the principles of the Amanpuri Diet, individuals can create a sustainable and healthy lifestyle that supports their health goals.

Whole Foods

Eating whole foods can be an effective way to support weight loss and hormonal control. Whole foods are nutrient-dense, unprocessed, and free from added sugars, preservatives, and artificial flavors, making them an ideal choice for those looking to maintain a healthy weight and balance their hormones. Here are some whole foods that can support weight loss and hormonal control:

- **Leafy Greens:** Leafy greens are a nutrient-dense food that can support weight loss and hormonal balance. Greens like spinach, kale, and collard greens are rich in vitamins, minerals, and fiber, which can help regulate hormones and improve digestion. They also contain antioxidants that help protect cells from damage.

- ☒ **Fatty Fish:** Fatty fish like salmon, tuna, and mackerel are a good source of omega-3 fatty acids, which can help regulate hormones and support weight loss. Omega-3s also have anti-inflammatory properties that can help reduce inflammation and protect against chronic diseases.

- ☒ **Whole Grains:** Whole grains like quinoa, brown rice, and oats are rich in fiber, which can help promote weight loss and regulate hormones. Fiber helps to slow the absorption of carbohydrates, which can help stabilize blood sugar levels and reduce insulin resistance.

- **Nuts and Seeds:** Nuts and seeds are a great source of healthy fats, protein, and fiber, which can help support weight loss and hormonal balance. They are also rich in antioxidants and micronutrients like magnesium and zinc, which are essential for hormonal health.

⊠ **Berries:** Berries like blueberries, strawberries, and raspberries are low-calorie, nutrient-dense food that can support weight loss and hormonal control. They are high in antioxidants, vitamins, and fiber, which can help reduce inflammation and improve digestion.

⊠ **Cruciferous Vegetables:** Cruciferous vegetables like broccoli, cauliflower, and Brussels sprouts are a good source of fiber and antioxidants, which can help support weight loss and hormonal balance. They also contain compounds called glucosinolates, which are thought to have anti-cancer properties.

☒ **Avocado:** Avocado is a healthy fat source that can support weight loss and hormonal control. It is rich in monounsaturated fats, fiber, and potassium, which can help regulate blood sugar levels and improve hormonal health.

☒ **Legumes:** Legumes like lentils, chickpeas, and black beans are a good source of protein, fiber, and micronutrients like iron and magnesium, which are essential for hormonal health. They can also help promote feelings of fullness and reduce cravings, which can support weight loss.

☒ **Lean Proteins:** Lean proteins like chicken, turkey, and tofu are a good source of high-quality protein, which can help support weight loss and hormonal control. Protein can also help regulate appetite and support muscle mass, which can help maintain a healthy weight.

■ **Fermented Foods:** Fermented foods like kimchi, sauerkraut, and kefir are rich in probiotics, which can support gut health and hormonal balance. A healthy gut microbiome is essential for hormonal health and weight loss.

Incorporating whole foods into your diet can be an effective way to support weight loss and hormonal control. By choosing nutrient-dense foods like leafy greens, fatty fish, whole grains, nuts and seeds, berries, cruciferous vegetables, avocado, legumes, lean proteins, and fermented foods, you can create a balanced and healthy diet that supports your overall health and well-being.

Low-Glycemic Index Foods

Low-GI foods are those that release glucose into the bloodstream at a slower rate, resulting in a more gradual and sustained increase in blood sugar levels. The glycemic index measures how quickly and how much a particular food raises blood glucose levels compared to pure glucose, which is assigned a value of 100. Foods with a lower GI value are generally considered to be more beneficial for blood sugar control and overall health.

The GI value of a food can vary depending on several factors, including the processing method, cooking method, and ripeness of the food. Generally, foods that are minimally processed and have a higher fiber content tend to have a lower GI. For example, an apple has a lower GI than apple juice because the apple contains more fiber.

Low-GI foods are also typically nutrient-dense, meaning they provide a high amount of nutrients per calorie. For example, whole grains are a good source of fiber, B vitamins, and minerals, such as iron and magnesium. Fruits and vegetables are rich in vitamins, minerals, and antioxidants that help protect the body against damage from free radicals.

When selecting low-GI foods, it is important to consider the glycemic load (GL) as well. The GL takes into account both the GI of the food and the number of carbohydrates in the food. Some foods with a high GI may have a low GL if they are consumed in small amounts, while some low-GI foods may have a high GL if they are consumed in large amounts. For example, watermelon has a high GI, but a low GL because it contains a small number of carbohydrates per serving.

Low-GI foods are typically rich in fiber, protein, and healthy fats, and are known to provide sustained energy and promote satiety, making them ideal for weight management and diabetes management. Here are some examples of low-GI foods:

1. Whole Grains: Whole grains, such as barley, quinoa, oats, and brown rice, are excellent sources of complex carbohydrates and fiber, which slow down the absorption of glucose into the bloodstream. They also provide a host of other nutrients, including B vitamins, iron, and magnesium.

2. Legumes: Legumes, such as lentils, chickpeas, and kidney beans, are rich

in protein, fiber, and complex carbohydrates, which promote sustained energy and slow the release of glucose into the bloodstream.

3. Fruits: Fruits, such as apples, pears, berries, and citrus fruits, are low in GI due to their high fiber and water content. They are also packed with vitamins, minerals, and antioxidants, making them a nutritious addition to any diet.

4. Vegetables: Non-starchy vegetables, such as leafy greens, broccoli, and cauliflower, are high in fiber and low in calories and carbohydrates, making

them an ideal choice for weight management and blood sugar control.

5. Nuts and Seeds: Nuts and seeds, such as almonds, walnuts, chia seeds, and flaxseeds, are high in healthy fats, protein, and fiber, which promote satiety and slow the release of glucose into the bloodstream.

6. Dairy: Low-fat dairy products, such as milk, yogurt, and cheese, are low in GI and provide a good source of protein, calcium, and vitamin D, which are important for bone health.

Consuming low-GI foods has been associated with a range of health benefits, including improved blood sugar control, reduced risk of type 2 diabetes, improved cardiovascular health, and weight management. However, it is important to note that the GI value of a food can be influenced by various factors, such as processing, cooking, and ripeness, and should be used as a guide rather than a definitive measure of a food's impact on blood sugar levels.

Healthy Fats

Fat is an essential nutrient for the body, and consuming the right types of fat can be beneficial for weight loss and hormonal control. Healthy fats provide the body with energy, support cell growth, and help to protect the organs. In this response, we will explore some of the best sources of healthy fats and how they can support weight loss and hormonal balance.

Avocado: Avocados are a great source of healthy fats, including monounsaturated and polyunsaturated fats. They are also rich in fiber, vitamins, and minerals. Eating avocado can help to promote feelings of fullness and can support weight loss efforts. Additionally, the healthy fats in avocados can help to regulate hormones and support healthy reproductive function.

Nuts and Seeds: Nuts and seeds, such as almonds, walnuts, chia seeds, and flaxseeds, are packed with healthy fats, fiber, and protein. These nutrients can help to promote feelings of fullness, support muscle growth, and aid in weight loss efforts. Nuts and seeds are also good sources of plant-based omega-3 fatty acids, which can help to reduce inflammation and support healthy hormone balance.

Olive Oil: Olive oil is a great source of monounsaturated fats, which can help to lower cholesterol levels and improve heart health. It can also help to regulate insulin levels and support weight loss efforts. Using olive oil as a substitute for butter or margarine can help to reduce overall calorie intake and promote weight loss.

Fatty Fish: Fatty fish, such as salmon, sardines, and tuna, are high in omega-3 fatty acids, which can help to reduce inflammation and support healthy hormone balance. These fats can also help to improve heart health, support brain function, and aid in weight loss efforts.

Coconut Oil: Coconut oil is a source of medium-chain triglycerides (MCTs), which are a type of fat that the body can quickly convert into energy. Consuming coconut oil can help to increase feelings of fullness and support weight loss efforts. It can also support healthy hormone balance and improve thyroid function.

Incorporating these healthy fats into the diet can be beneficial for weight loss and hormonal balance. However, it is important to consume them in moderation and to balance them with other important nutrients, such as protein and fiber. Additionally, it is important to choose healthy fat sources and to avoid consuming too many saturated and trans fats, which can be harmful to overall health.

Adequate Protein

Adequate protein intake is essential for weight loss and hormonal control. Protein is one of the three macronutrients, along with carbohydrates and fats, and it plays a critical role in many bodily functions. Protein is essential for building and repairing tissues, including muscle, skin, and bones, and it is also involved in hormone production and regulation.

When it comes to weight loss, consuming adequate protein can help to promote satiety and reduce cravings, which can aid in calorie control. Protein also has a higher thermic effect than carbohydrates or fats, which means that the body burns more calories digesting and processing protein than it does digest and processing other nutrients.

In addition to aiding in weight loss, adequate protein intake is important for hormonal control. Protein is necessary for the production of hormones, including insulin, glucagon, and growth hormone. These hormones play a critical role in regulating metabolism, blood sugar levels, and muscle growth and repair.

The amount of protein needed varies depending on factors such as age, sex, and activity level. The Recommended Dietary Allowance (RDA) for protein is 0.8 grams per kilogram of body weight per day. However, for individuals who are trying to lose weight or maintain muscle mass, a higher protein intake may be beneficial.

Some good sources of protein include lean meats, such as chicken, turkey, and beef, as well as fish, eggs, dairy products, and plant-based sources, such as legumes, nuts, and seeds. It is important to choose protein sources that are low in saturated and trans fats and to incorporate a variety of protein sources into the diet.

Here are some additional details about the benefits of protein for weight loss and hormonal control:

- ⊠ **Promotes satiety**: Protein is a satiating macronutrient that can help to reduce hunger and promote feelings of fullness. This is because protein slows down the rate at which the stomach empties and stimulates the release of hormones that signal fullness to the brain. As a result, consuming adequate protein can help to reduce overall calorie intake, which is beneficial for weight loss.

- **Preserves muscle mass:** When losing weight, it is important to preserve muscle mass to maintain metabolic rate and prevent weight regain. Adequate protein intake can help to preserve muscle mass, especially when combined with resistance training. This is because protein is necessary for muscle protein synthesis, which is the process by which the body builds new muscle tissue.

⊠ **Supports hormonal balance:** Adequate protein intake is necessary for the production of hormones, such as insulin, glucagon, and growth hormone. These hormones play a critical role in regulating metabolism, blood sugar levels, and muscle growth and repair. Consuming adequate protein can help to support hormonal balance and prevent hormonal imbalances that can lead to weight gain and other health issues.

⊠ **Improves metabolic rate:** Protein has a higher thermic effect than carbohydrates or fats, which means that the body burns more calories digesting and processing protein than it does digest and processing other nutrients. This increased energy expenditure can lead to a higher metabolic rate, which is beneficial for weight loss and weight management.

In conclusion, adequate protein intake is essential for weight loss and hormonal control. Protein can promote satiety, preserve muscle mass, support hormonal balance, and improve metabolic rate. To achieve optimal health, it is important to consume a balanced diet that includes a variety of nutrient-dense protein sources.

Avoiding Processed Foods and Sugar

Avoiding processed foods and sugar is an important part of a healthy diet for weight loss and hormonal control. Processed foods are often high in calories, unhealthy fats, sugar, and sodium, and they provide little to no nutritional value. Consuming too much sugar can lead to hormonal imbalances, inflammation, and weight gain.

Here are some reasons why avoiding processed foods and sugar is beneficial for weight loss and hormonal control:

- ☒ **Reduced calorie intake**: Processed foods are often high in calories and low in nutrients, which can lead to overconsumption and weight gain. By avoiding processed foods and choosing whole, nutrient-dense foods instead, you can reduce your overall calorie intake and promote weight loss.

⊠ **Reduced sugar intake:** Consuming too much sugar can lead to hormonal imbalances, inflammation, and weight gain. Processed foods are often high in added sugars, which can contribute to these negative health effects. By avoiding processed foods and sugary drinks, you can reduce your sugar intake and improve hormonal balance.

⊠ **Improved insulin sensitivity:** Insulin is a hormone that regulates blood sugar levels, and insulin resistance is a common precursor to type 2 diabetes and other metabolic disorders. Consuming too much sugar and processed foods can lead to insulin resistance while avoiding these foods can improve insulin sensitivity and reduce the risk of these conditions.

☒ **Reduced inflammation:** Processed foods and sugar can contribute to inflammation in the body, which is associated with a variety of health issues, including obesity, insulin resistance, and cardiovascular disease. By avoiding these foods, you can reduce inflammation and promote overall health.

To avoid processed foods and sugar, focus on consuming whole, nutrient-dense foods, such as fruits, vegetables, whole grains, lean proteins, and healthy fats. Avoid processed snacks, sugary drinks, and desserts, and limit your intake of packaged foods that are high in sodium, unhealthy fats, and added sugars.

Avoiding processed foods and sugar is an important part of a healthy diet for weight loss and hormonal control. By focusing on whole, nutrient-dense foods and limiting your intake of processed foods and sugar, you can promote overall health and improve your chances of reaching and maintaining a healthy weight.

CHAPTER FOUR

Sample Meal Plan for weight loss and hormonal control

A sample meal plan for weight loss and hormonal control should focus on nutrient-dense, whole foods that provide a balance of protein, healthy fats, and complex carbohydrates. Here is an example of a one-day meal plan:

Breakfast:

2 boiled eggs

1 cup of cooked spinach

1 slice of whole grain toast with avocado spread

Snack:

1 small apple

1 tbsp almond butter

Lunch:

Grilled chicken breast

1 cup of roasted sweet potatoes

1 cup of sautéed broccoli

1 tbsp of olive oil

Snack:

1 cup of sliced cucumbers and carrots

1/4 cup of hummus

Dinner:

Grilled salmon fillet

1 cup of quinoa

1 cup of roasted Brussels sprouts

1 tbsp of avocado oil

Dessert:

1 small bowl of mixed berries with 1/4 cup of Greek yogurt

This sample meal plan provides a balance of protein, healthy fats, and complex carbohydrates throughout the day. It also includes plenty of nutrient-dense fruits and vegetables to provide vitamins and minerals.

Here are some key features of this meal plan:

- ☒ Protein is included in every meal and snack to promote satiety and preserve muscle mass.

- ☒ Healthy fats are incorporated through foods like avocado, almond butter, olive oil, and salmon to support hormonal balance.

- ☒ Complex carbohydrates are included in foods like sweet potatoes, quinoa, and whole-grain toast to provide sustained energy and fiber.

- ☒ Snacks are included to prevent overeating at meals and to provide additional nutrients throughout the day.

- ☒ Dessert is included in moderation to satisfy cravings without overindulging in sugar.

Remember, a meal plan should be tailored to individual needs and preferences, so this is just one example. It is important to work with a healthcare professional or registered dietitian to develop a personalized meal plan that meets your specific needs and goals.

Here are 28 sample meal plans for weight loss and hormonal control, each providing a balance of protein, healthy fats, and complex carbohydrates:

Meal Plan 1:

Breakfast: Scrambled eggs with spinach and mushrooms, 1 slice of whole grain toast with avocado spread

Snack: Small apple with 1 tbsp almond butter

Lunch: Grilled chicken breast with mixed greens salad, 1/4 avocado, and 1 tbsp balsamic vinaigrette

Snack: Carrots and celery with hummus

Dinner: Grilled salmon with roasted sweet potatoes and asparagus

Dessert: Greek yogurt with mixed berries

Meal Plan 2:

Breakfast: Greek yogurt with mixed berries and almonds

Snack: Pear with 1 oz cheddar cheese

Lunch: Turkey burger with lettuce wrap, sliced tomatoes, and sweet potato fries

Snack: Sliced cucumbers with guacamole.

Dinner: Grilled chicken kebab with mixed greens salad and 1 tbsp olive oil and lemon juice dressing

Dessert: Dark chocolate with almonds

Meal Plan 3:

Breakfast: Oatmeal with mixed berries, almonds, and 1 tbsp almond butter

Snack: Banana with 1 tbsp peanut butter

Lunch: Grilled shrimp with mixed greens salad, 1/4 avocado, and 1 tbsp honey mustard dressing

Snack: Celery and cherry tomatoes with hummus

Dinner: Grilled salmon with roasted Brussels sprouts and quinoa

Dessert: Baked apple with cinnamon and 1 tbsp Greek yogurt

Meal Plan 4:

Breakfast: Egg and vegetable scramble with 1 slice of whole-grain toast

Snack: Peach with 1 oz almonds

Lunch: Grilled chicken breast with mixed greens salad, 1/4 avocado, and 1 tbsp vinaigrette

Snack: Sliced cucumber with tzatziki sauce

Dinner: Grilled flank steak with roasted sweet potatoes and green beans

Dessert: 1/2 cup Greek yogurt with 1/2 cup mixed berries

Meal Plan 5:

Breakfast: Greek yogurt with mixed berries and walnuts

Snack: Orange with 1 oz cheddar cheese

Lunch: Grilled shrimp with mixed greens salad, 1/4 avocado, and 1 tbsp balsamic vinaigrette

Snack: Carrots and celery with ranch dressing

Dinner: Grilled salmon with roasted asparagus and quinoa

Dessert: Dark chocolate with cashews

Meal Plan 6:

Breakfast: Omelet with spinach, mushrooms, and feta cheese

Snack: Apple with 1 tbsp almond butter

Lunch: Turkey wrap with lettuce, sliced tomatoes, and 1/2 avocado

Snack: Sliced cucumbers with tzatziki sauce

Dinner: Grilled chicken with roasted sweet potatoes and green beans

Dessert: Baked pear with cinnamon and 1 tbsp Greek yogurt

Meal Plan 7:

Breakfast: Egg and vegetable scramble with 1 slice of whole-grain toast

Snack: Peach with 1 oz almonds

Lunch: Grilled chicken breast with mixed greens salad, 1/4 avocado, and 1 tbsp vinaigrette

Snack: Sliced cucumber with hummus

Dinner: Grilled salmon with roasted Brussels sprouts and quinoa

Dessert: 1/2 cup Greek yogurt with 1/2 cup mixed berries

Meal Plan 8:

Breakfast: Greek yogurt with mixed berries and pistachios

Snack: Small apple with 1 oz cheddar cheese

Lunch: Grilled chicken breast with mixed greens salad, 1/4 avocado, and 1 tbsp honey mustard dressing

Snack: Carrots and cherry tomatoes with hummus

Dinner: Grilled salmon with roasted sweet potatoes and green beans

Dessert: Baked apple with cinnamon and 1 tbsp Greek yogurt

Meal Plan 9:

Breakfast: Omelet with spinach, mushrooms, and 1 slice of whole grain toast

Snack: Orange with 1 oz almonds

Lunch: Turkey burger with lettuce wrap, sliced tomatoes, and sweet potato fries

Snack: Sliced cucumbers with guacamole

Dinner: Grilled flank steak with roasted Brussels sprouts and quinoa

Dessert: Dark chocolate with cashews

Meal Plan 10:

Breakfast: Scrambled eggs with spinach and mushrooms, 1 slice of whole grain toast with avocado spread

Snack: Pear with 1 tbsp almond butter

Lunch: Grilled shrimp with mixed greens salad, 1/4 avocado, and 1 tbsp vinaigrette

Snack: Celery and cherry tomatoes with ranch dressing

Dinner: Grilled chicken with roasted sweet potatoes and asparagus

Dessert: Greek yogurt with mixed berries and walnuts

Meal Plan 11:

Breakfast: Oatmeal with mixed berries, almonds, and 1 tbsp almond butter

Snack: Banana with 1 tbsp peanut butter

Lunch: Grilled chicken breast with mixed greens salad, 1/4 avocado, and 1 tbsp balsamic vinaigrette

Snack: Sliced cucumber with tzatziki sauce

Dinner: Grilled salmon with roasted Brussels sprouts and quinoa

Dessert: Baked pear with cinnamon and 1 tbsp Greek yogurt

Meal Plan 12:

Breakfast: Greek yogurt with mixed berries and cashews

Snack: Small apple with 1 oz cheddar cheese

Lunch: Grilled chicken breast with mixed greens salad, 1/4 avocado, and 1 tbsp honey mustard dressing

Snack: Carrots and celery with hummus

Dinner: Grilled flank steak with roasted sweet potatoes and green beans

Dessert: Dark chocolate with pistachios

Meal Plan 13:

Breakfast: Egg and vegetable scramble with 1 slice of whole-grain toast

Snack: Orange with 1 oz almonds

Lunch: Turkey wrap with lettuce, sliced tomatoes, and 1/2 avocado

Snack: Sliced cucumbers with guacamole

Dinner: Grilled salmon with roasted asparagus and quinoa

Dessert: Baked apple with cinnamon and 1 tbsp Greek yogurt

Meal Plan 14:

Breakfast: Oatmeal with mixed berries, walnuts, and 1 tbsp almond butter

Snack: Banana with 1 tbsp peanut butter

Lunch: Grilled shrimp with mixed greens salad, 1/4 avocado, and 1 tbsp balsamic vinaigrette

Snack: Celery and cherry tomatoes with ranch dressing

Dinner: Grilled chicken with roasted sweet potatoes and green beans

Dessert: Greek yogurt with mixed berries and pistachios

Meal Plan 15:

Breakfast: Spinach and mushroom omelet with 1 slice of whole-grain toast

Snack: Apple slices with 1 tbsp almond butter

Lunch: Grilled chicken breast with mixed greens salad, 1/4 avocado, and 1 tbsp honey mustard dressing

Snack: Carrots and cherry tomatoes with hummus

Dinner: Grilled salmon with roasted Brussels sprouts and quinoa

Dessert: Dark chocolate with pistachios

Meal Plan 16:

Breakfast: Greek yogurt with mixed berries and walnuts

Snack: Banana with 1 oz almonds

Lunch: Grilled shrimp with mixed greens salad, 1/4 avocado, and 1 tbsp vinaigrette

Snack: Sliced cucumber with tzatziki sauce

Dinner: Grilled chicken with roasted sweet potatoes and green beans

Dessert: Baked apple with cinnamon and 1 tbsp Greek yogurt

Meal Plan 17:

Breakfast: Oatmeal with mixed berries, almonds, and 1 tbsp almond butter

Snack: Small apple with 1 oz cheddar cheese

Lunch: Turkey burger with lettuce wrap, sliced tomatoes, and sweet potato fries

Snack: Sliced cucumbers with guacamole

Dinner: Grilled flank steak with roasted Brussels sprouts and quinoa

Dessert: Dark chocolate with cashews

Meal Plan 18:

Breakfast: Scrambled eggs with spinach and mushrooms, 1 slice of whole grain toast with avocado spread

Snack: Orange with 1 oz almonds

Lunch: Grilled chicken breast with mixed greens salad, 1/4 avocado, and 1 tbsp balsamic vinaigrette

Snack: Celery and cherry tomatoes with ranch dressing

Dinner: Grilled salmon with roasted asparagus and quinoa

Dessert: Greek yogurt with mixed berries and pistachios

Meal Plan 19:

Breakfast: Greek yogurt with mixed berries and cashews

Snack: Pear with 1 tbsp peanut butter

Lunch: Grilled chicken breast with mixed greens salad, 1/4 avocado, and 1 tbsp honey mustard dressing

Snack: Carrots and celery with hummus

Dinner: Grilled flank steak with roasted sweet potatoes and green beans

Dessert: Baked pear with cinnamon and 1 tbsp Greek yogurt

Meal Plan 20:

Breakfast: Oatmeal with mixed berries, walnuts, and 1 tbsp almond butter

Snack: Banana with 1 oz cheddar cheese

Lunch: Grilled shrimp with mixed greens salad, 1/4 avocado, and 1 tbsp balsamic vinaigrette

Snack: Sliced cucumber with tzatziki sauce

Dinner: Grilled chicken with roasted Brussels sprouts and quinoa

Dessert: Dark chocolate with pistachios

Meal Plan 21:

Breakfast: Egg and vegetable scramble with 1 slice of whole-grain toast

Snack: Apple slices with 1 tbsp almond butter

Lunch: Grilled chicken breast with mixed greens salad, 1/4 avocado, and 1 tbsp vinaigrette

Snack: Carrots and cherry tomatoes with hummus

Dinner: Grilled salmon with roasted sweet potatoes and asparagus

Dessert: Baked apple with cinnamon and 1 tbsp Greek yogurt.

Meal Plan 22:

Breakfast: Spinach and feta omelet with 1 slice of whole-grain toast
Snack: Pear with 1 oz cashews
Lunch: Grilled chicken breast with mixed greens salad, 1/4 avocado, and 1 tbsp honey mustard dressing
Snack: Sliced cucumber with tzatziki sauce
Dinner: Grilled salmon with roasted asparagus and quinoa

Dessert: Dark chocolate with pistachios

Meal Plan 23:

Breakfast: Greek yogurt with mixed berries and walnuts

Snack: Banana with 1 oz almonds

Lunch: Grilled chicken breast with mixed greens salad, 1/4 avocado, and 1 tbsp vinaigrette

Snack: Sliced bell peppers with hummus

Dinner: Grilled shrimp with roasted sweet potatoes and green beans

Dessert: Baked apple with cinnamon and 1 tbsp Greek yogurt

Meal Plan 24:

Breakfast: Oatmeal with mixed berries, almonds, and 1 tbsp almond butter

Snack: Small apple with 1 oz cheddar cheese

Lunch: Turkey burger with lettuce wrap, sliced tomatoes, and sweet potato fries

Snack: Carrots and celery with ranch dressing

Dinner: Grilled flank steak with roasted Brussels sprouts and quinoa

Dessert: Dark chocolate with cashews

Meal Plan 25:

Breakfast: Egg and vegetable scramble with 1 slice of whole-grain toast

Snack: Apple slices with 1 tbsp almond butter

Lunch: Grilled chicken breast with mixed greens salad, 1/4 avocado, and 1 tbsp balsamic vinaigrette

Snack: Carrots and cherry tomatoes with hummus

Dinner: Grilled salmon with roasted sweet potatoes and asparagus

Dessert: Baked pear with cinnamon and 1 tbsp Greek yogurt

Meal Plan 26:

Breakfast: Greek yogurt with mixed berries and pistachios

Snack: Orange with 1 oz almonds

Lunch: Grilled shrimp with mixed greens salad, 1/4 avocado, and 1 tbsp honey mustard dressing

Snack: Sliced cucumber with tzatziki sauce

Dinner: Grilled chicken with roasted Brussels sprouts and quinoa

Dessert: Dark chocolate with pistachios

Meal Plan 27:

Breakfast: Oatmeal with mixed berries, walnuts, and 1 tbsp almond butter

Snack: Pear with 1 oz cashews

Lunch: Grilled chicken breast with mixed greens salad, 1/4 avocado, and 1 tbsp vinaigrette

Snack: Sliced bell peppers with hummus

Dinner: Grilled salmon with roasted asparagus and quinoa

Dessert: Baked apple with cinnamon and 1 tbsp Greek yogurt

Meal Plan 28:

Breakfast: Spinach and mushroom omelet with 1 slice of whole-grain toast

Snack: Banana with 1 oz almonds

Lunch: Grilled chicken breast with mixed greens salad, 1/4 avocado, and 1 tbsp balsamic vinaigrette

Snack: Sliced cucumber with tzatziki sauce

Dinner: Grilled flank steak with roasted sweet potatoes and green beans

Dessert: Dark chocolate with cashews

CHAPTER FIVE

Supplements and Lifestyle Changes That Support Hormonal Balance and Weight Loss

Hormonal imbalances can make it difficult to lose weight and maintain healthy body composition. However, several supplements and lifestyle changes can help support hormonal balance and weight loss efforts.

Supplements:

Omega-3 fatty acids: Omega-3 fatty acids have been shown to help reduce inflammation and improve insulin sensitivity, which can help support hormonal balance and weight loss. They are commonly found in fatty fish like salmon and mackerel, but can also be taken as a supplement.

- **Vitamin D:** Vitamin D deficiency has been linked to hormonal imbalances and weight gain. Supplementing with vitamin D can help support healthy hormone levels and may aid in weight loss efforts.

☒ **Magnesium**: Magnesium plays a role in over 300 enzymatic reactions in the body, including those involved in hormone regulation. Supplementing with magnesium may help support hormonal balance and improve insulin sensitivity.

☒ **Probiotics**: The gut microbiome plays a crucial role in hormone production and metabolism. Taking a probiotic supplement can help support a healthy gut microbiome and may aid in weight loss efforts.

- ⊠ **Zinc**: Zinc is essential for the production and metabolism of hormones, including insulin, thyroid hormone, and testosterone. Supplementing with zinc may help support healthy hormone levels and improve weight loss efforts.

- ⊠ **Chromium**: Chromium is involved in insulin signaling and glucose metabolism, and supplementing with chromium may improve insulin sensitivity and support weight loss.

☒ **Green tea extract:** Green tea extract contains catechins, which have been shown to help support weight loss by increasing metabolism and fat oxidation.

☒ **Fiber supplements**: Increasing fiber intake has been shown to help support weight loss and improve insulin sensitivity. Taking a fiber supplement like psyllium husk can help increase fiber intake and support healthy hormone levels.

Lifestyle changes:

- ☒ **Exercise**: Regular exercise can help support hormonal balance and aid in weight loss efforts. Strength training is particularly effective at increasing muscle mass and reducing body fat, which can help improve insulin sensitivity and support healthy hormone levels.

- **Sleep**: Adequate sleep is crucial for hormone regulation and weight loss. Aim for 7-9 hours of sleep per night to support healthy hormone levels and improve weight loss efforts.

- **Stress management**: Chronic stress can hurt hormone balance and weight loss. Incorporating stress-reducing activities like yoga, meditation, or deep breathing into your daily routine can help support healthy hormone levels and improve weight loss efforts.

- **Balanced nutrition:** Eating a balanced diet that is rich in whole foods, healthy fats, and protein can help support hormonal balance and weight loss. Avoiding processed foods and sugar can also help reduce inflammation and support healthy hormone levels.

- **Limiting alcohol and caffeine:** Excessive alcohol and caffeine intake can disrupt hormone balance and interfere with weight loss efforts. Limiting alcohol and caffeine consumption may help support healthy hormone levels and improve weight loss efforts.

❌ **Mindful eating:** Practicing mindful eating can help improve hormone balance and support weight loss efforts. Mindful eating involves paying attention to hunger and fullness cues, eating slowly, and savoring the flavors and textures of food.

❌ **Hydration**: Drinking plenty of water can help support healthy hormone levels and aid in weight loss efforts. Aim for at least 8 glasses of water per day.

☒ **Time-restricted eating:** Time-restricted eating involves limiting the window of time during which you consume food. This can help improve insulin sensitivity and support weight loss efforts. For example, you may choose to only eat during an 8-hour window each day, such as from 10 am to 6 pm.

☒ **Reduce exposure to endocrine disruptors**: Endocrine disruptors are chemicals found in certain plastics, pesticides, and personal care products that can interfere with hormone balance. Reducing exposure to these chemicals can help support healthy hormone levels and aid in weight loss efforts.

By incorporating a combination of these supplements and lifestyle changes into your daily routine, you can support hormonal balance and improve your weight loss efforts.

However, it's important to remember that everyone's body is different, and what works for one person may not work for another. It's always recommended to work with a healthcare professional to develop a personalized plan that is right for you.

In conclusion, supporting hormonal balance and weight loss efforts requires a holistic approach that includes both supplements and lifestyle changes. By incorporating these strategies into your daily routine, you may be able to improve your hormonal balance and achieve your weight loss goals. However, it is always recommended to consult with a healthcare professional before making any significant changes to your diet or supplement regimen.

Stress Management

Stress is a common factor that can negatively impact both weight loss efforts and hormonal balance. Stress can cause an increase in the hormone cortisol, which can lead to increased appetite, cravings for high-calorie foods, and fat storage. Additionally, stress can disrupt sleep, which can further exacerbate hormonal imbalances.

Managing stress is crucial for maintaining hormonal balance and supporting weight loss efforts. Here are some stress management techniques that can help:

- ☒ **Exercise**: Exercise is a great way to manage stress, as it releases endorphins, which are natural mood-boosting chemicals. Exercise can also help regulate hormone levels and support weight loss efforts.

- ☒ **Mind–body techniques**: Mind-body techniques such as yoga, meditation, and deep breathing can help reduce stress and improve hormone balance. These techniques can help activate the relaxation response, which can reduce cortisol levels and support weight loss efforts.

- ☒ **Adequate sleep:** Getting enough sleep is essential for supporting hormonal balance and weight loss efforts. Aim for 7-9 hours of sleep per night to support healthy hormone levels and reduce stress.

- ☒ **Social support:** Having a support system can help reduce stress and improve hormone balance. Connect with friends, family, or a support group to help manage stress and support your weight loss efforts.

- ☒ **Time management:** Effective time management can help reduce stress and improve hormone balance. Prioritize tasks, delegate when possible, and avoid over-committing to help reduce stress levels.

☒ **Relaxation techniques:** Relaxation techniques such as taking a warm bath, listening to calming music, or spending time in nature can help reduce stress and support weight loss efforts.

By incorporating stress management techniques into your daily routine, you can support hormonal balance and improve your weight loss efforts. However, it's important to remember that everyone's body is different, and what works for one person may not work for another. It's always recommended to work with a healthcare professional to develop a personalized plan that is right for you.

CHAPTER SIX

Tips for Success on the Amanpuri Diet

The Amanpuri diet is a low-glycemic, anti-inflammatory diet that focuses on whole foods and healthy fats. Here are ten tips for success on the Amanpuri diet:

Plan: Plan out your meals and snacks ahead of time to ensure that you have healthy options available throughout the day.

Focus on whole foods: Choose whole foods such as vegetables, fruits, nuts, seeds, lean proteins, and healthy fats.

Avoid processed foods: Avoid processed foods that are high in sugar, refined carbohydrates, and unhealthy fats.

Include healthy fats: Incorporate healthy fats such as olive oil, avocado, nuts, and seeds into your meals and snacks.

Eat low-glycemic foods: Choose low-glycemic foods such as non-starchy vegetables, berries, and legumes to help balance blood sugar levels.

Limit high-glycemic foods: Limit high-glycemic foods such as refined carbohydrates, sugary drinks, and processed snacks.

Include protein at every meal: Incorporate protein such as chicken, fish, tofu, or beans at every meal to help keep you feeling full and satisfied.

Drink plenty of water: Aim to drink at least 8 glasses of water per day to stay hydrated and support weight loss efforts.

Practice mindful eating: Eat slowly, savor your food, and pay attention to your hunger and fullness cues to help prevent overeating.

Incorporate physical activity: Incorporate regular physical activity into your daily routine to help support weight loss efforts and overall health.

Plan your meals: Take the time to plan your meals, including snacks, so that you always have healthy options on hand. Use the Amanpuri Diet guidelines to create a balanced meal plan that includes plenty of whole foods.

Stock up on healthy foods: Make sure your pantry and fridge are stocked with healthy options like fruits, vegetables, lean proteins, and whole grains. This will make it easier to stick to your diet plan and avoid temptation.

Stay hydrated: Drinking plenty of water is essential for good health and weight loss. Aim to drink at least 8 glasses of water per day, and consider adding herbal tea or lemon water to your routine for added flavor and benefits.

Get moving: Exercise is an important part of any weight loss plan. Incorporate regular physical activity into your routine, such as walking, running, swimming, or yoga.

Get support: Enlist the help of friends or family members who can provide support and encouragement as you work towards your weight loss goals. Consider joining a support group or working with a registered dietitian or personal trainer.

Stay positive: Losing weight can be challenging, but maintaining a positive attitude can help keep you motivated and on track. Celebrate your successes along the way, and don't get discouraged by setbacks or plateaus.

Be patient: Remember that weight loss is a journey, and it may take time to see results. Focus on making sustainable lifestyle changes that you can maintain over the long term.

Track your progress: Keep track of your weight loss progress and celebrate your milestones along the way. Consider using a food diary or a tracking app to help you stay accountable.

Focus on overall health: Remember that the Amanpuri Diet is not just about weight loss, but about improving overall health and well-being. Focus on nourishing your body with whole, nutrient-dense foods, and enjoy the benefits of improved energy, mood, and vitality.

By following these tips, you can successfully follow the Amanpuri diet and achieve your weight loss and health goals. However, it's important to remember that everyone's body is different, and what works for one person may not work for another. It's always recommended to work with a healthcare professional to develop a personalized plan that is right for you.

CHAPTER SEVEN

Conclusion

Summary of the Amanpuri Diet

The Amanpuri Diet is a nutrition plan that emphasizes whole, nutrient-dense foods to improve health and promote weight loss. It is based on the principles of the Mediterranean diet, with an emphasis on lean proteins, whole grains, fruits, vegetables, and healthy fats like olive oil and nuts. The diet recommends avoiding processed foods, sugar, and refined carbohydrates. It also emphasizes mindful eating and regular physical activity to support overall health and well-being. The Amanpuri Diet is designed to be sustainable and can be customized to fit individual needs and preferences.

Here are some additional details about the Amanpuri Diet:

The Amanpuri Diet is based on the Mediterranean diet: The Mediterranean diet is known for its health benefits, including improved heart health, better weight management, and lower risk of chronic diseases. The Amanpuri Diet incorporates many of the same principles, such as a focus on whole foods and healthy fats.

It emphasizes whole, nutrient-dense foods: The Amanpuri Diet encourages eating a variety of whole, nutrient-dense foods, such as fruits, vegetables, whole grains, lean proteins, and healthy fats. These foods are rich in vitamins, minerals, and fiber, and can help support overall health and well-being.

It recommends avoiding processed foods: The Amanpuri Diet recommends avoiding processed foods, sugar, and refined carbohydrates. These foods can contribute to inflammation, weight gain, and other health issues.

It emphasizes mindful eating: The Amanpuri Diet encourages mindful eating, which means paying attention to your hunger and fullness cues, savoring your food, and avoiding distractions like TV or your phone. This can help you eat more slowly, appreciate your food more, and avoid overeating.

It recommends regular physical activity: The Amanpuri Diet emphasizes the importance of regular physical activity for overall health and weight loss. Exercise can help improve heart health, boost metabolism, and promote feelings of well-being.

It can be customized to fit individual needs: The Amanpuri Diet is flexible and can be customized to fit individual needs and preferences. For example, vegetarians or vegans can follow the plan by incorporating plant-based protein sources, and those with food allergies or intolerances can adjust the plan accordingly.

It is designed to be sustainable: The Amanpuri Diet is designed to be a sustainable lifestyle change, rather than a short-term diet. By focusing on whole, nutrient-dense foods and regular physical activity, the plan can help individuals achieve long-term weight loss and improve overall health and well-being.

Overall, the Amanpuri Diet emphasizes the importance of eating whole, nutrient-dense foods and engaging in regular physical activity for improved health and weight loss. By making sustainable lifestyle changes, individuals can achieve long-term success and maintain a healthy weight and well-being.

Potential Results of Following the Amanpuri Diet

Following the Amanpuri Diet has the potential to yield several health benefits, including weight loss, improved heart health, and better blood sugar control. Here are some potential results of following the Amanpuri Diet:

Weight loss: The Amanpuri Diet emphasizes whole, nutrient-dense foods and regular physical activity, both of which can support weight loss. By eating fewer processed foods and sugar and consuming more fiber-rich foods and healthy fats, individuals may experience a reduction in body weight and body fat percentage.

Improved heart health: The Amanpuri Diet is rich in heart-healthy foods like fruits, vegetables, whole grains, and healthy fats. These foods are low in saturated fat and can help reduce cholesterol levels and lower the risk of heart disease. Additionally, regular physical activity can help improve heart health and reduce the risk of heart disease.

Better blood sugar control: The Amanpuri Diet emphasizes eating foods that are low on the glycemic index, meaning they don't cause a rapid spike in blood sugar levels. This can help improve blood sugar control and reduce the risk of type 2 diabetes.

Increased energy and improved mood: The Amanpuri Diet focuses on nutrient-dense foods that provide sustained energy throughout the day. Eating a balanced diet and engaging in regular physical activity can also help improve mood and reduce stress.

Improved digestion: The Amanpuri Diet emphasizes whole foods that are high in fiber, which can help support healthy digestion and prevent constipation.

Reduced inflammation: The Amanpuri Diet recommends avoiding processed foods and sugar, which can contribute to inflammation in the body. Eating a diet rich in whole, nutrient-dense foods and healthy fats can help reduce inflammation and improve overall health.

Following the Amanpuri Diet has the potential to yield a variety of health benefits, including weight loss, improved heart health, better blood sugar control, increased energy and improved mood, improved digestion, and reduced inflammation.

Final Thoughts and Recommendations.

Weight loss and hormonal control are two interconnected aspects of overall health and well-being. Here are some final thoughts and recommendations for achieving both:

Focus on nutrient-dense foods: Eating a diet that is rich in whole, nutrient-dense foods can help support both weight loss and hormonal balance. Foods like fruits, vegetables, whole grains, lean proteins, and healthy fats provide the vitamins, minerals, and nutrients that your body needs to function optimally.

Avoid processed foods and sugar: Processed foods and sugar can contribute to inflammation, insulin resistance, and hormonal imbalances, all of which can make it harder to lose weight and maintain hormonal balance. Avoiding these foods and choosing whole foods instead can help improve both weight loss and hormonal control.

Engage in regular physical activity: Regular physical activity can help support weight loss, reduce stress, and improve hormonal balance. Aim for at least 30 minutes of moderate-intensity exercise most days of the week.

Get enough sleep: Sleep plays a crucial role in hormonal control, with inadequate sleep being associated with insulin resistance and weight gain. Aim for at least 7-8 hours of sleep per night to support hormonal balance and weight loss.

Manage stress: Chronic stress can disrupt hormonal balance and make it harder to lose weight. Practicing stress-management techniques like meditation, deep breathing, or yoga can help support both hormonal control and weight loss.

In summary, achieving weight loss and hormonal control requires a holistic approach that focuses on whole, nutrient-dense foods, regular physical activity, adequate sleep, and stress management. By incorporating these strategies into your daily routine, you can support both weight loss and hormonal balance and achieve optimal health and well-being.